# Anatomy Urogenital System Label Practice

By K.R. Lefkowitz
Copyright © 2016 K.R. Lefkowitz

All rights reserved.
ISBN: 10:1533001375
ISBN-13: 978-1533001375

1. BREAST
2. FEMALE REPRODUCTIVE 1
3. FEMALE REPRODUCTIVE 2
4. FEMALE REPRODUCTIVE INTERNAL
5. FEMALE REPRODUCTIVE & FETUS
6. KIDNEY - EXTERIOR
7. KIDNEY - INTERIOR
8. KIDNEY- INTERIOR
9. KIDNEYS IN SITU 1
10. KIDNEYS IN SITU 2
11. KIDNEYS IN SITU 3
12. MALE REPRODUCTION 1
13. MALE REPRODUCTION 2
14. MAMARY- MUSCULATURE
15. MAMMARY
16. OVARY & UTERINE TUBE
17. PELVIS - FEMALE
18. PELVIS - MALE
19. PELVIS & PERINEUM - FEMALE
20. PELVIS & PERINEUM - MALE
21. PERINEUM - FEMALE
22. PERINEUM - MALE
23. RENAL CORPUSCLE
24. URINARY SYSTEM
25. UROGENITAL SYSTEM - MALE
26. UTERUS, OVARIES & LIGAMENTS

# How To Use....

This book is mean't to be used for you to label and practice the components of the muscular system. In going through your anatomy class and later in medical field you will need to know how to label the components, pictures of each system and know it inside and out. The best way is for you to label all the components that you know yourself and research the areas that you don't. Can you label all parts of the muscles, both deep and superficial, Urogenital system etc...? Can you recognize a picture and know immediately what it is? You can find the corresponding picture in the table of contents. Nothing is labeled on purpose. This is for you to label. For you to know. And what you don't know for you to research in your texts and find the answers. Through this way of learning and researching the parts you don't know, allows you to actually learn it and have it stored in long term memory. This active way of learning will in the long term be beneficial beyond belief in your future career or knowledge. Mark the pages, make notes, and use this practice book and pictures to help you understand the parts of the anatomy.

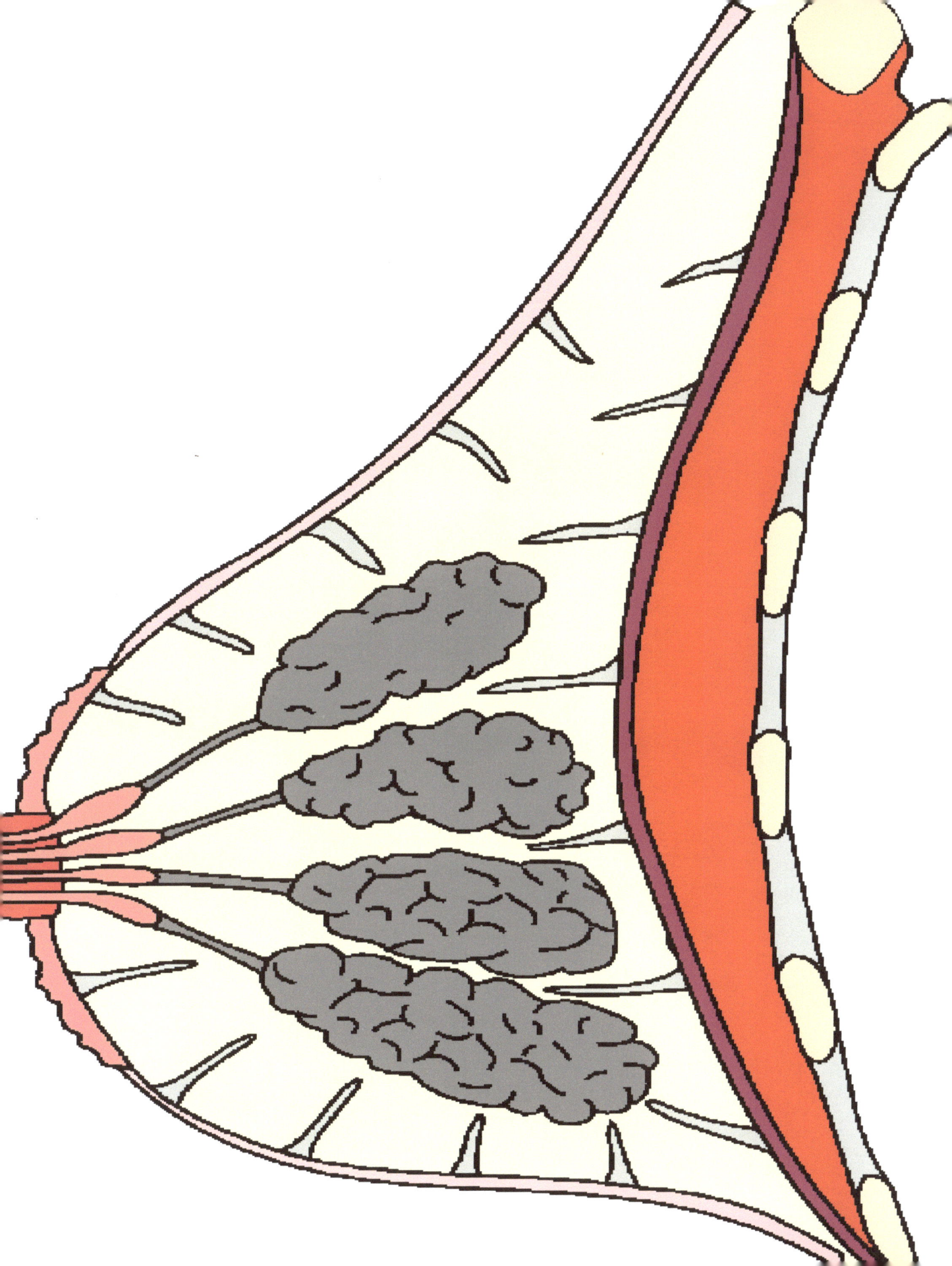

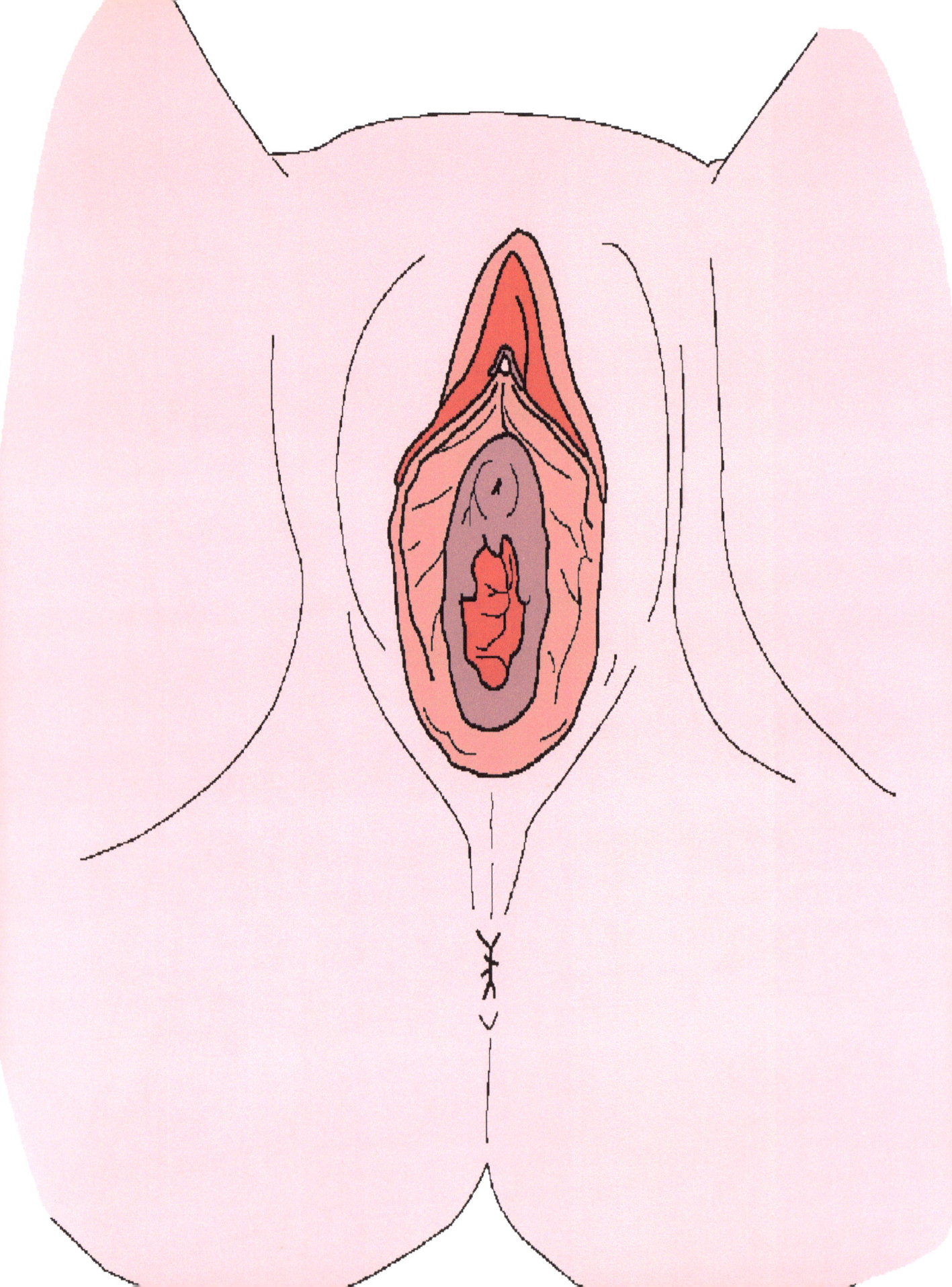

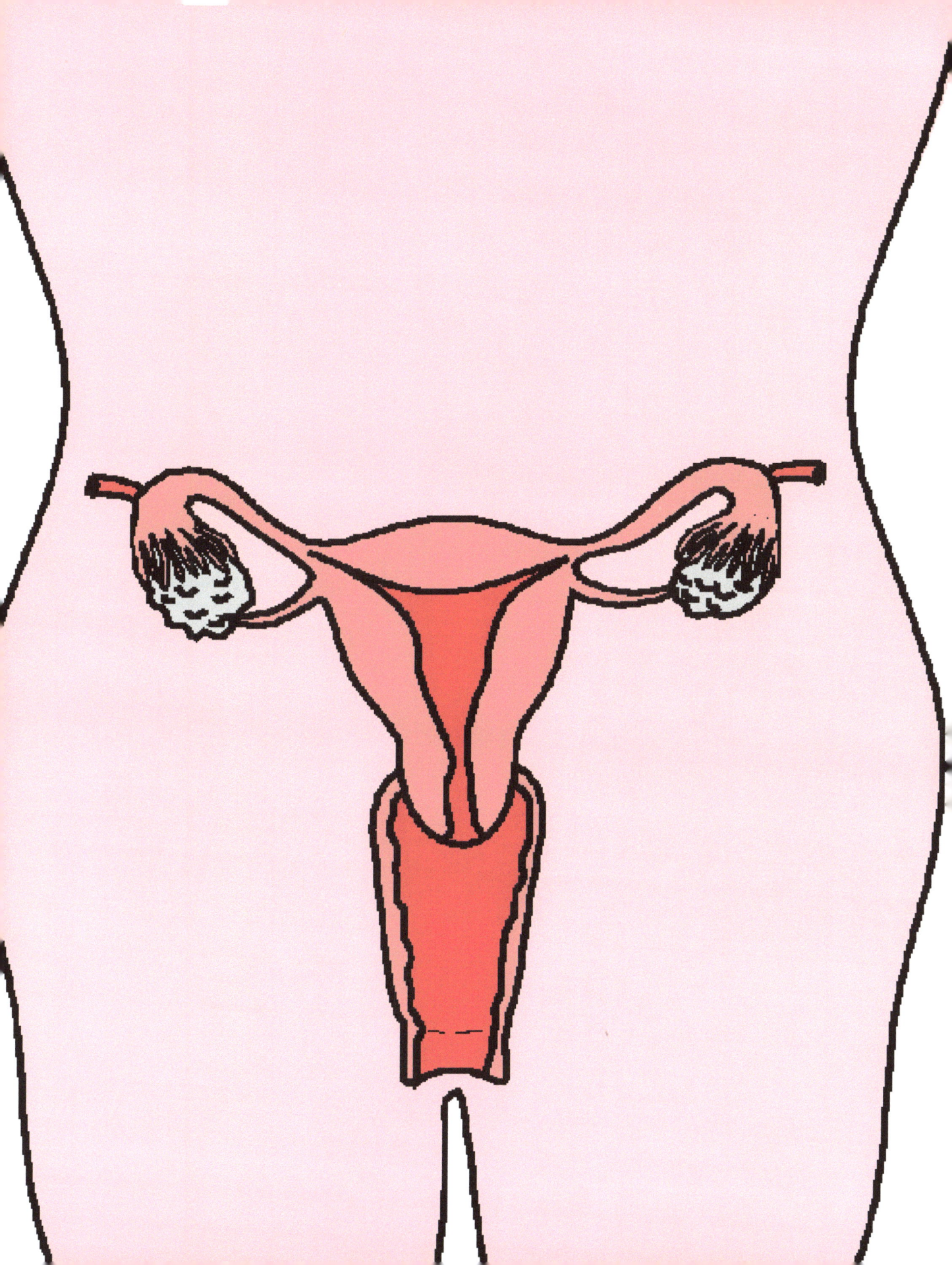

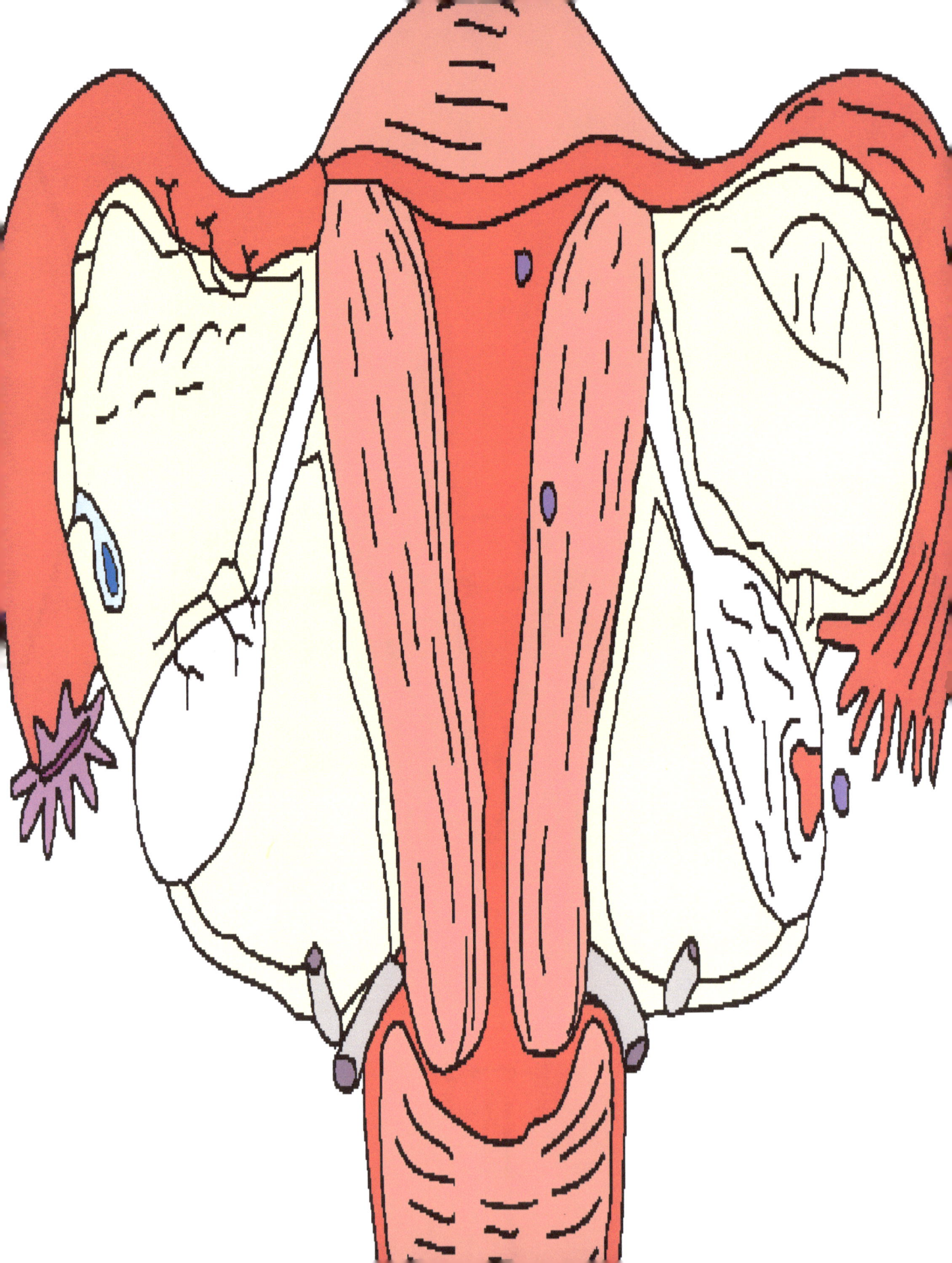

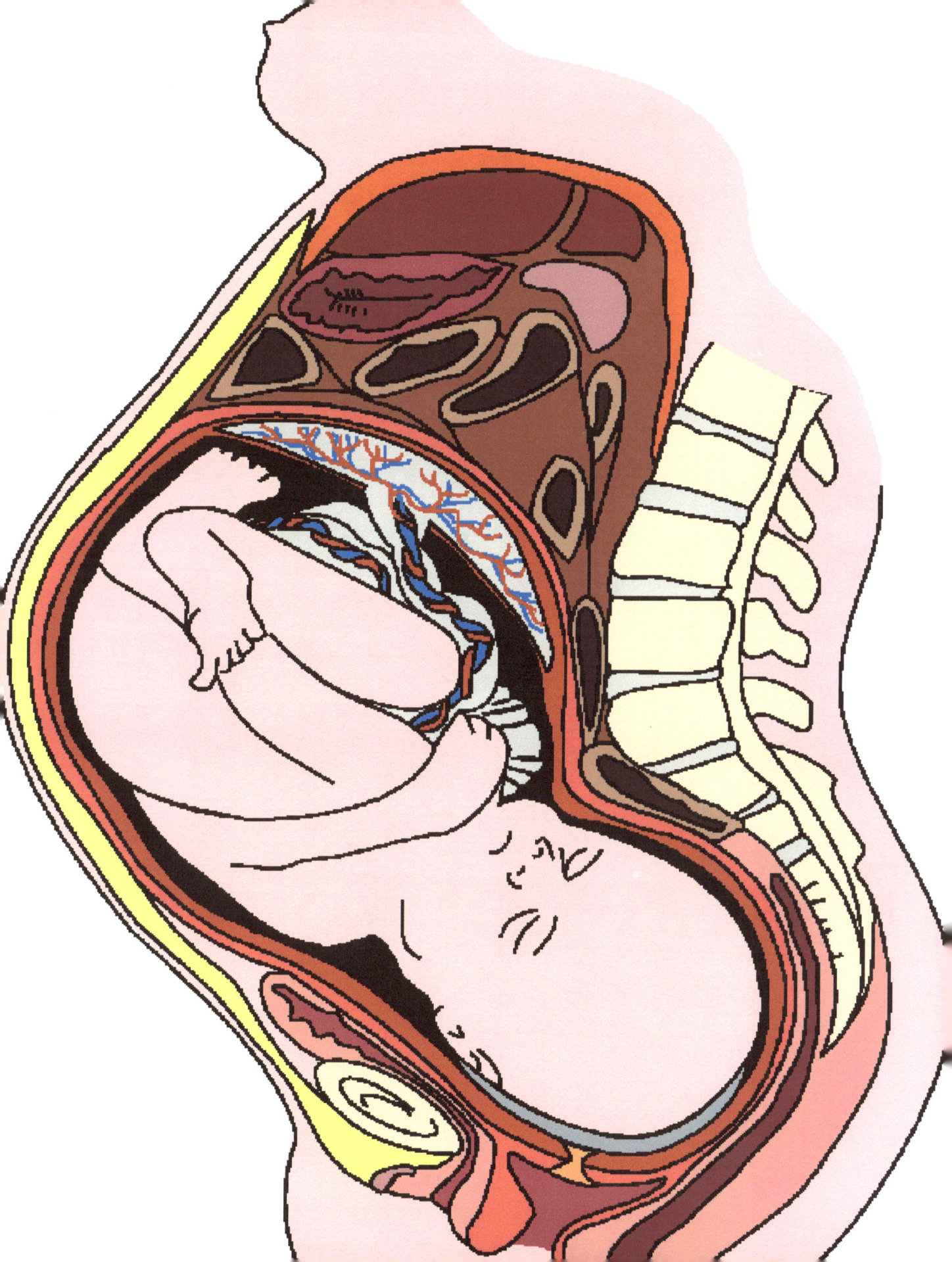

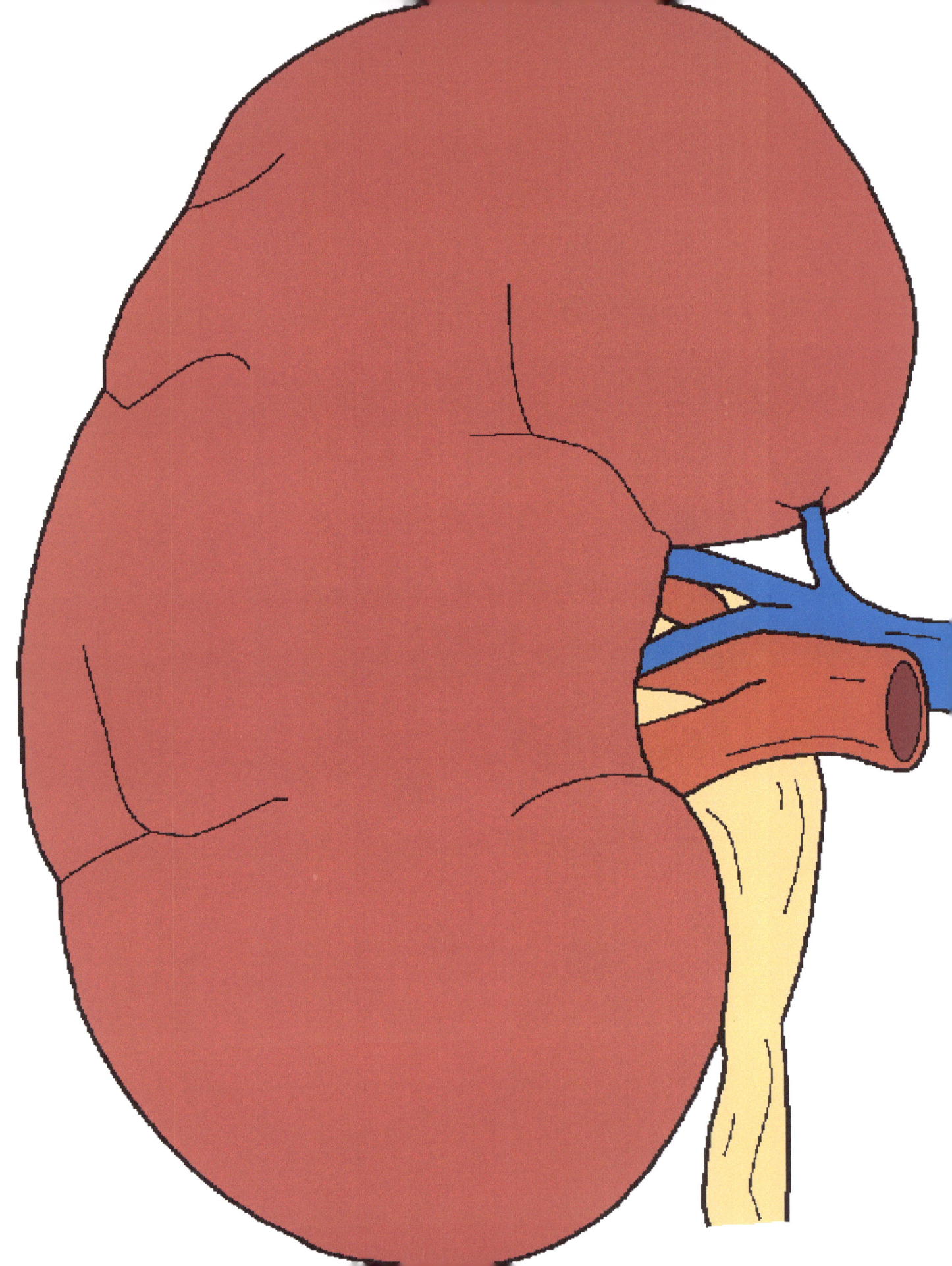

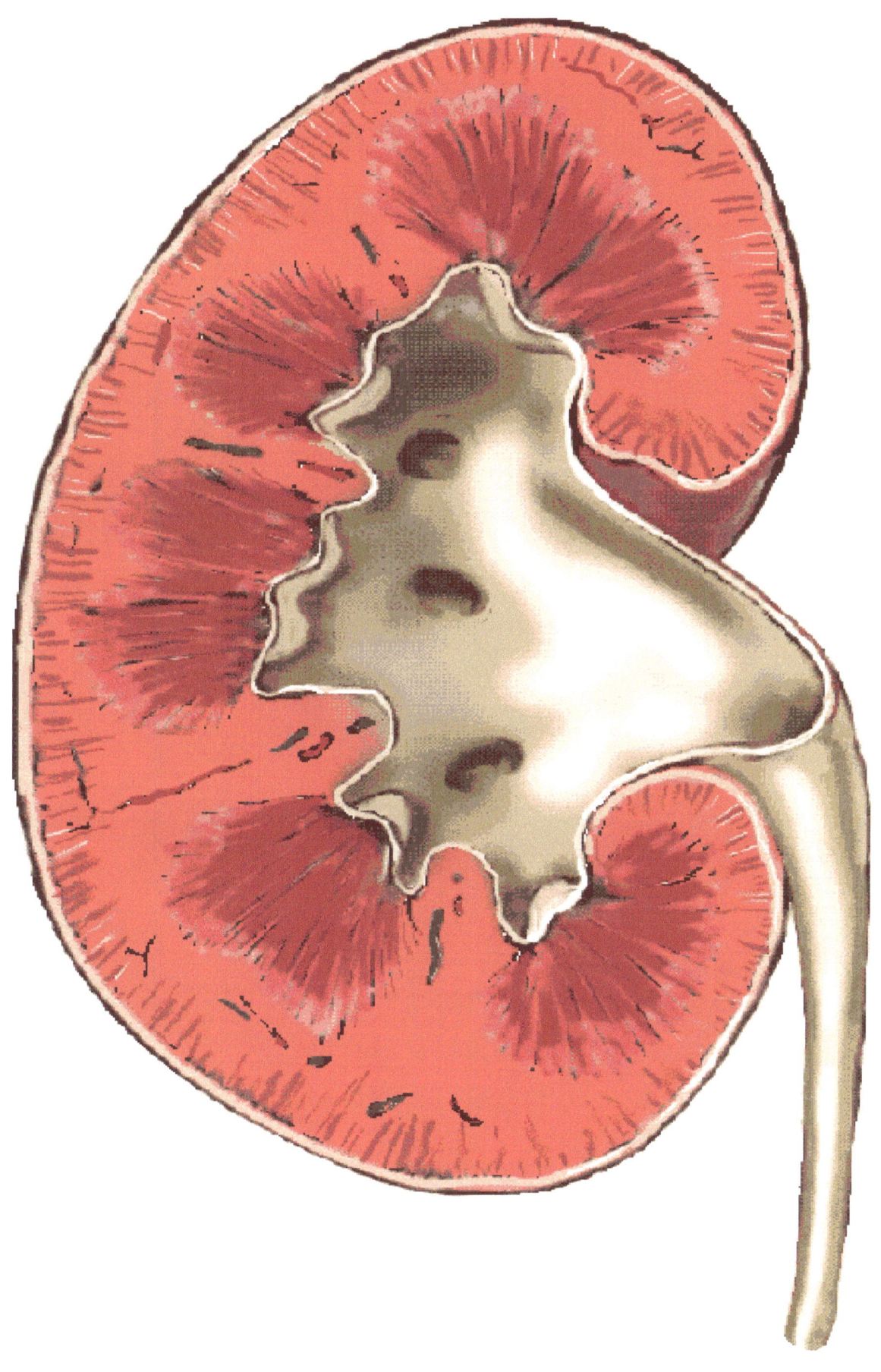

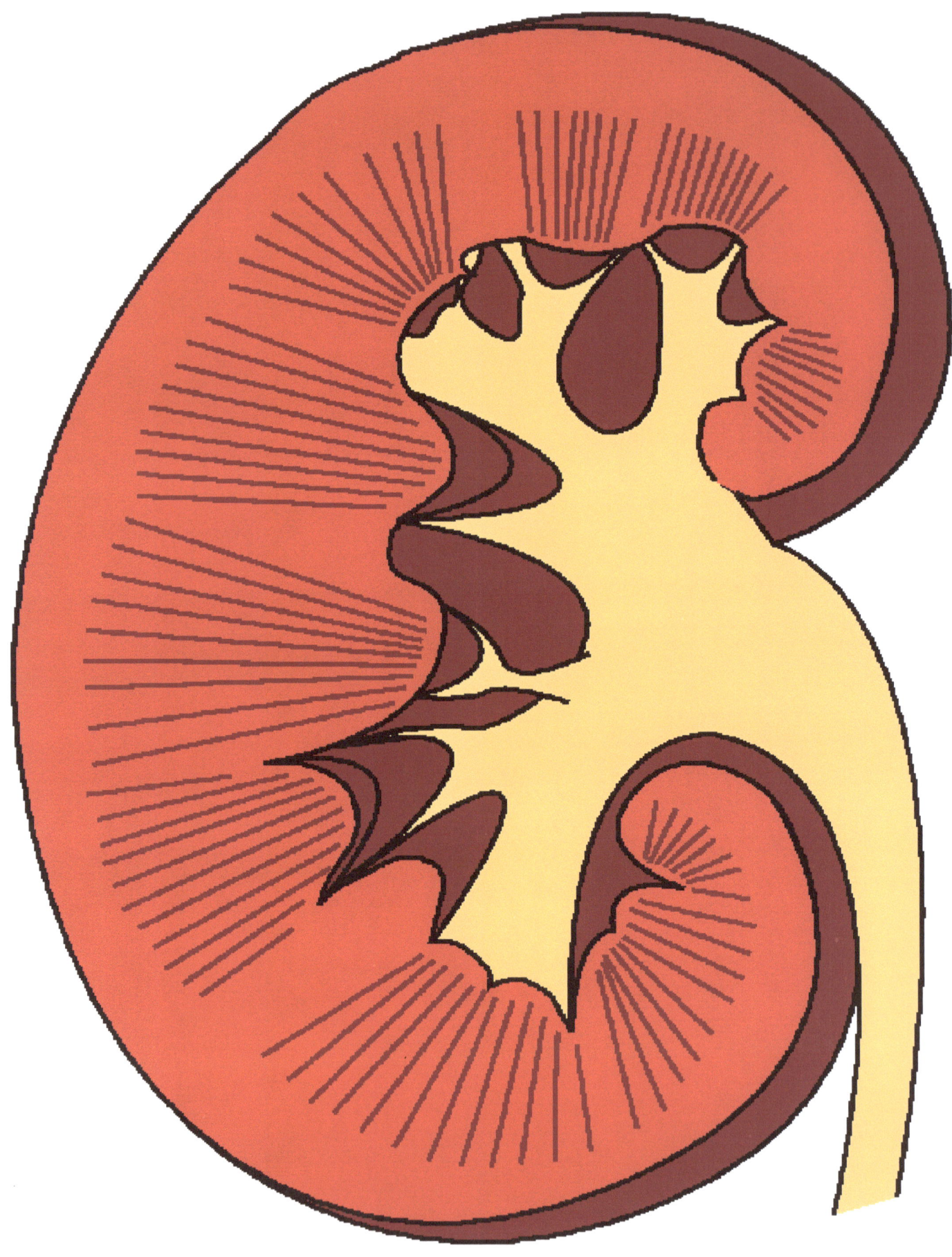

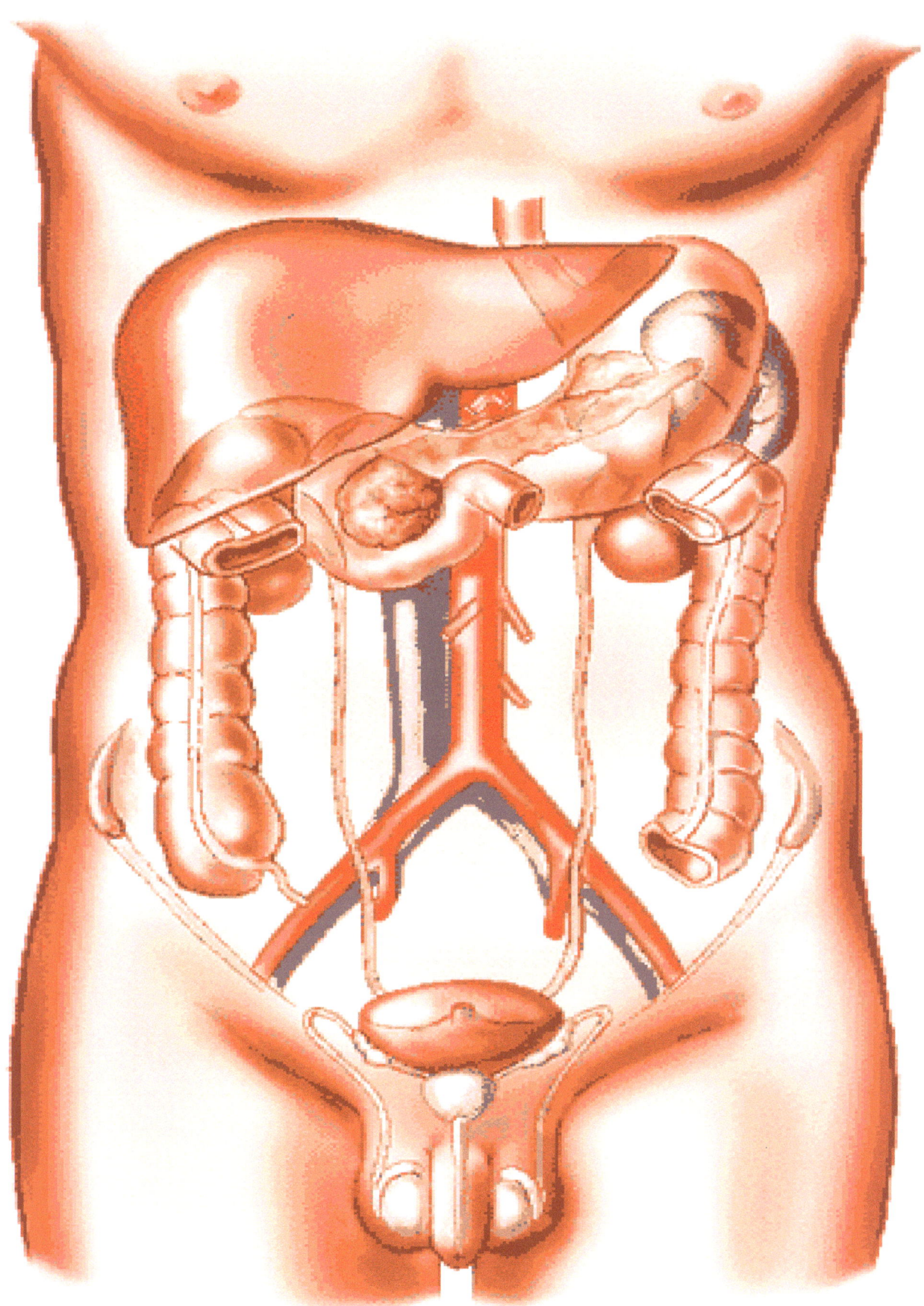

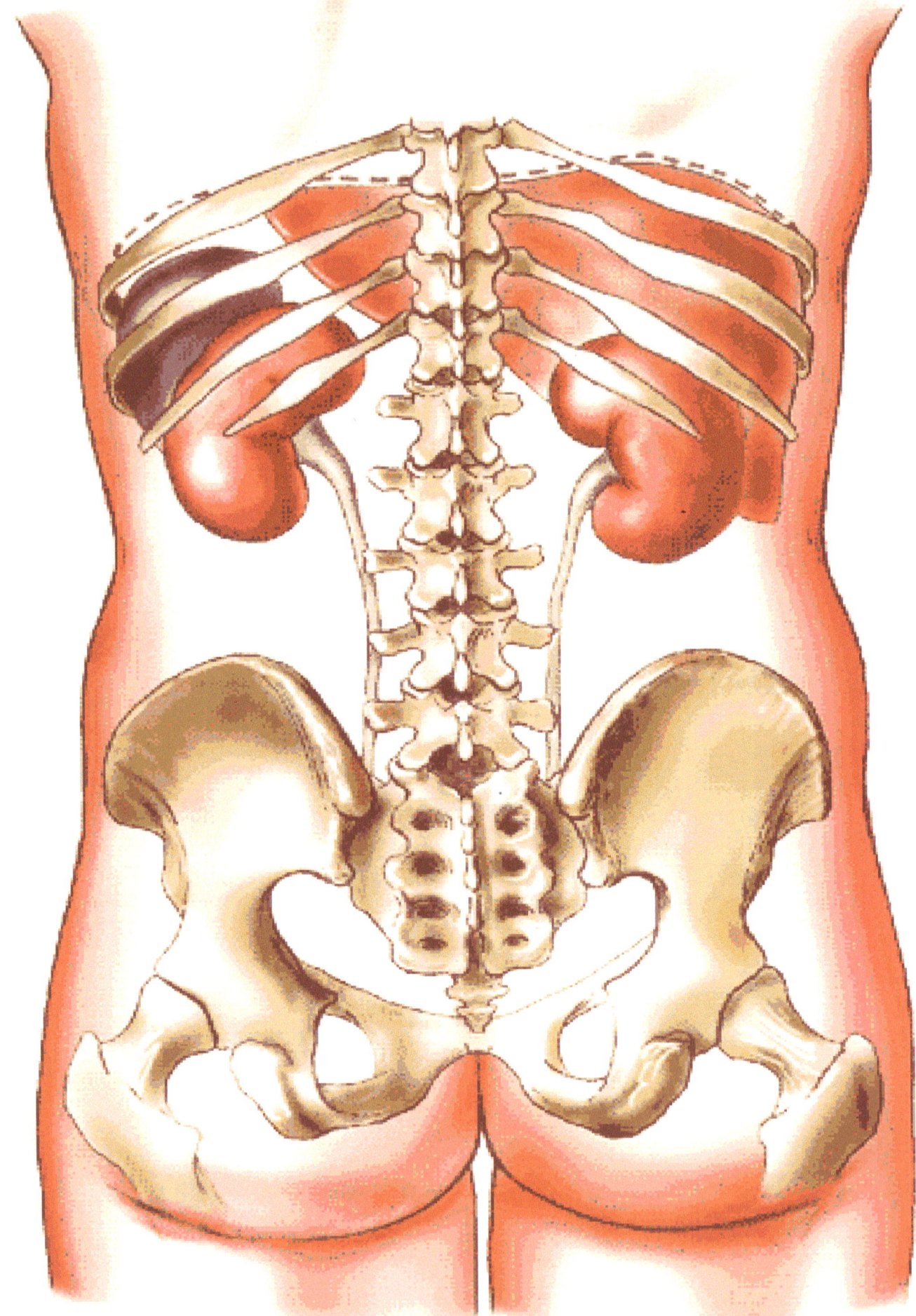

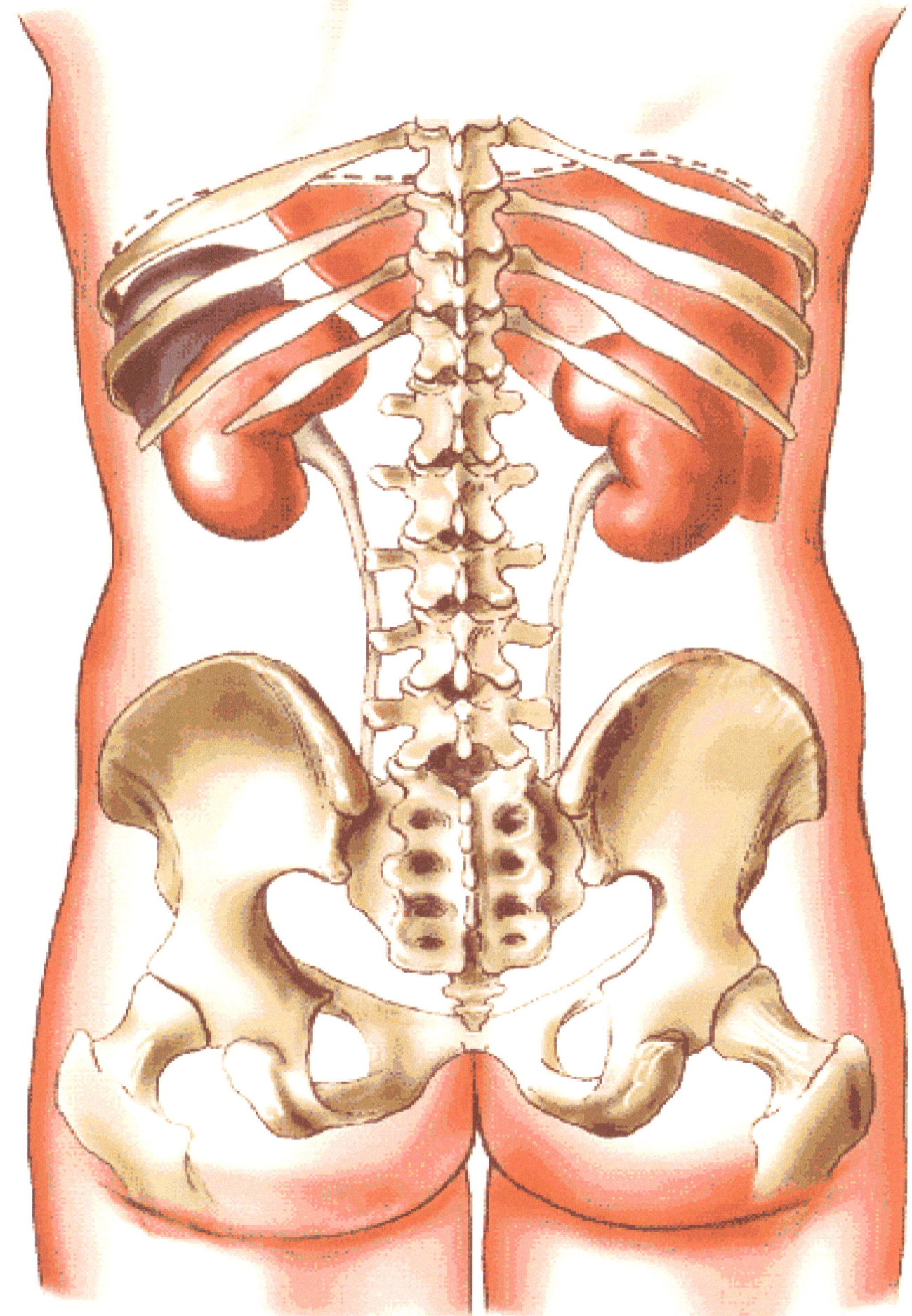

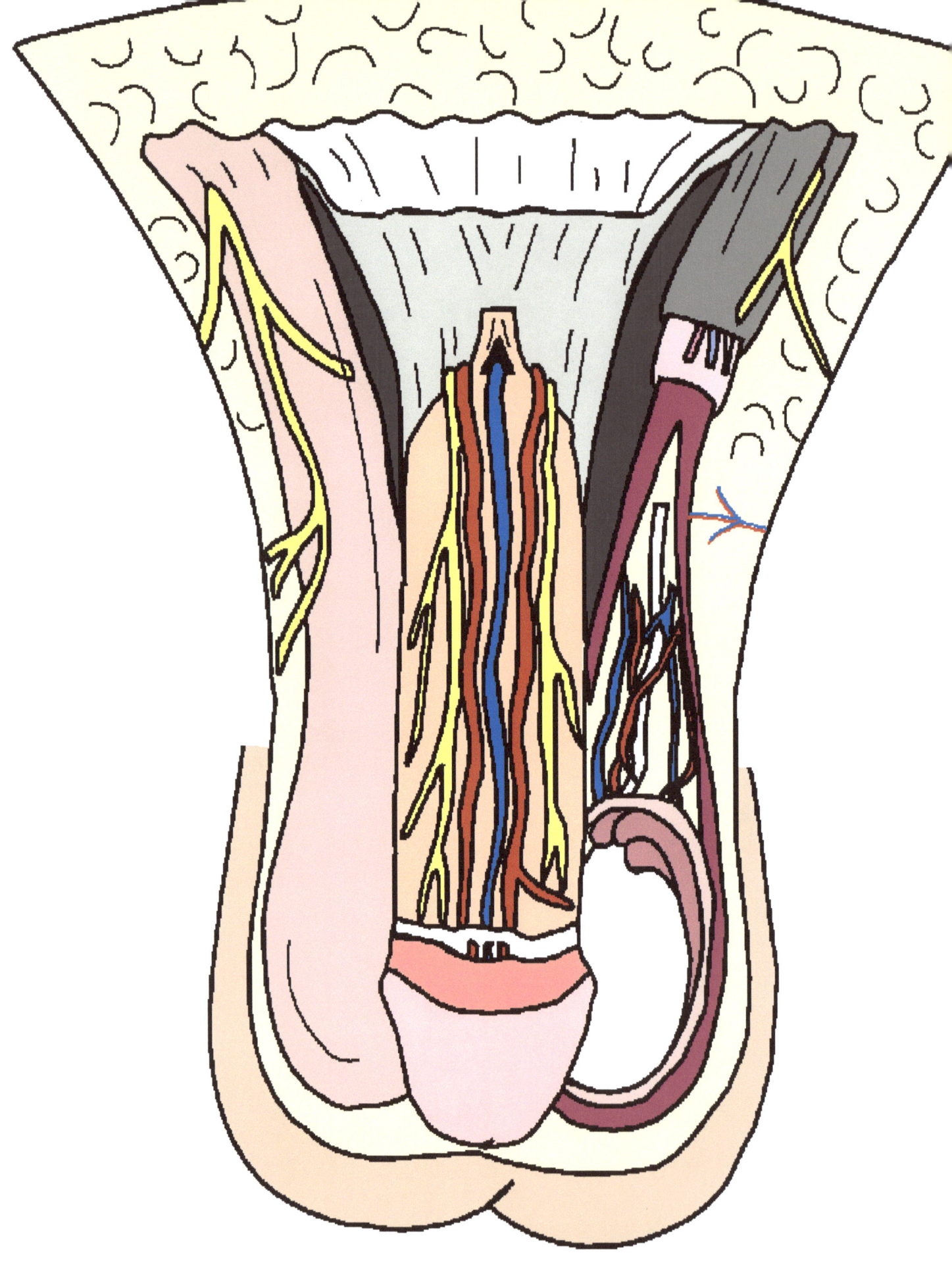

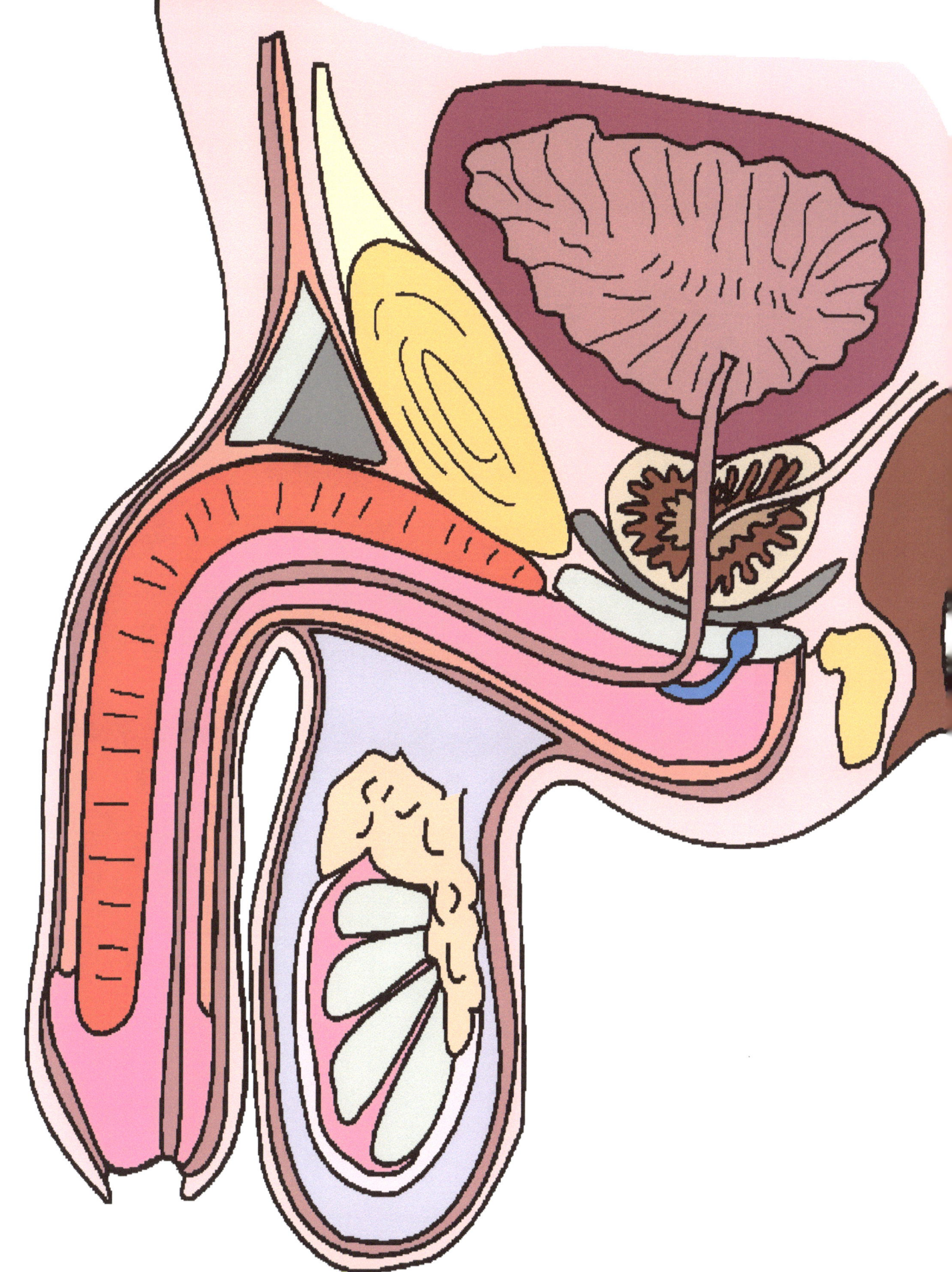

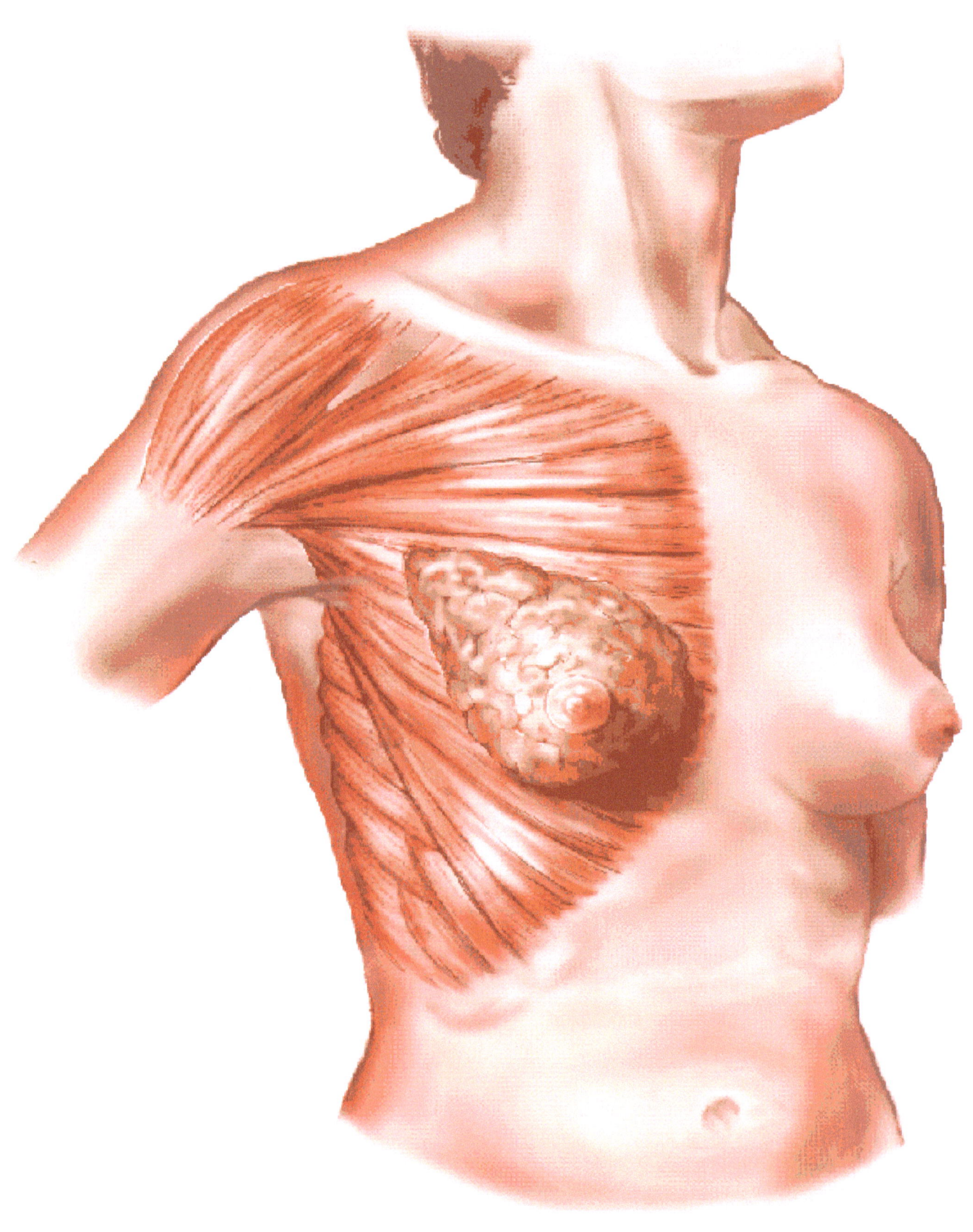

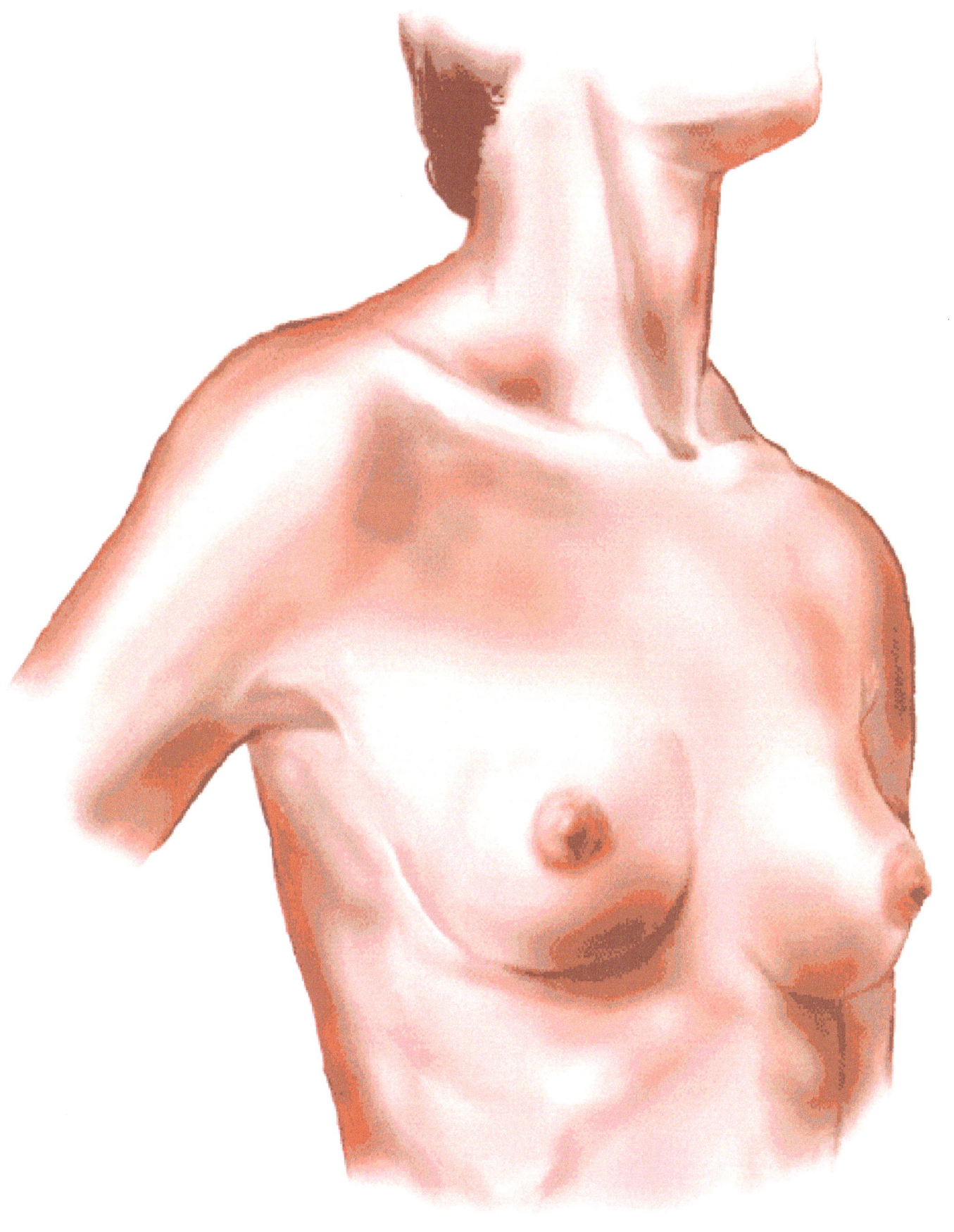

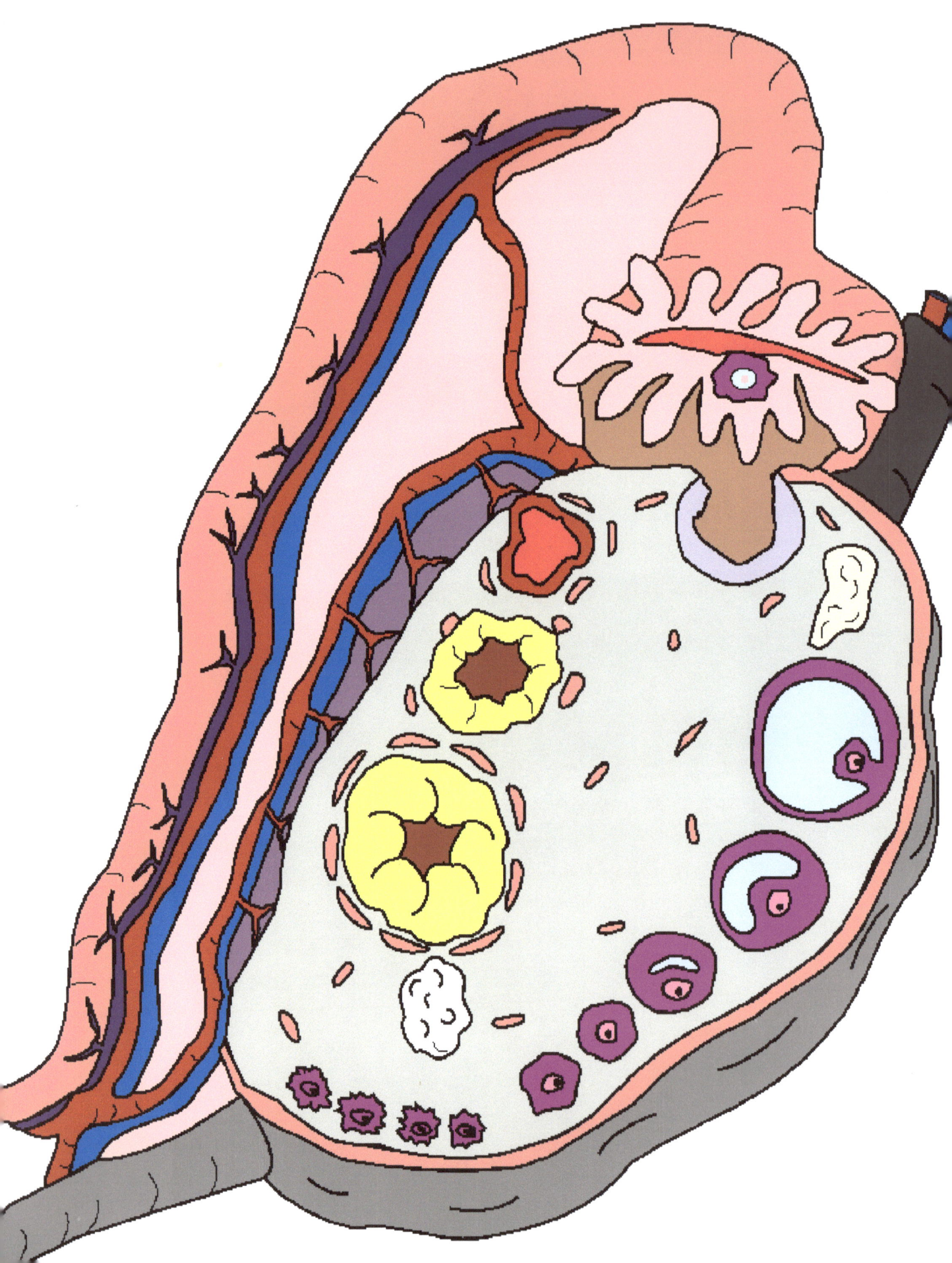

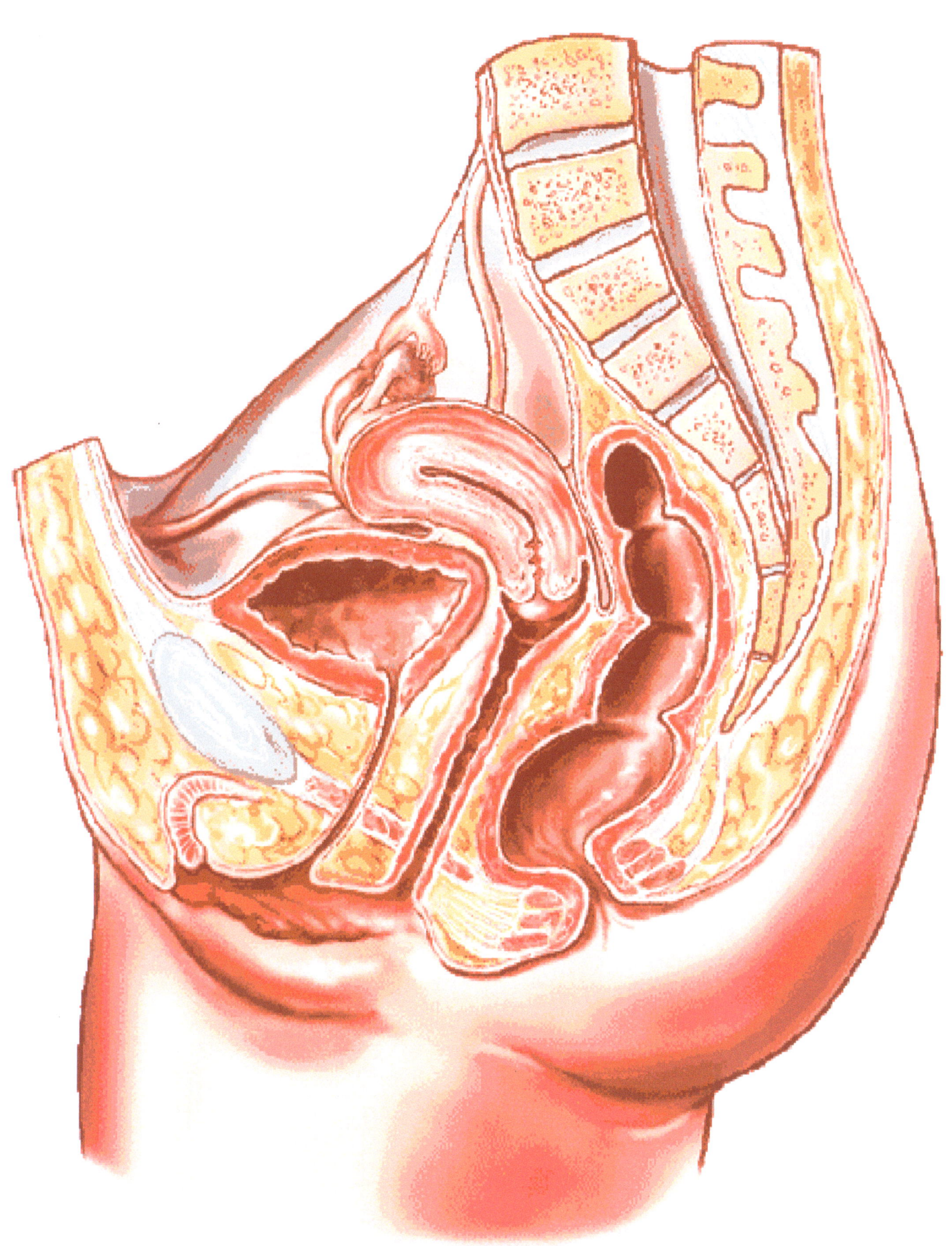

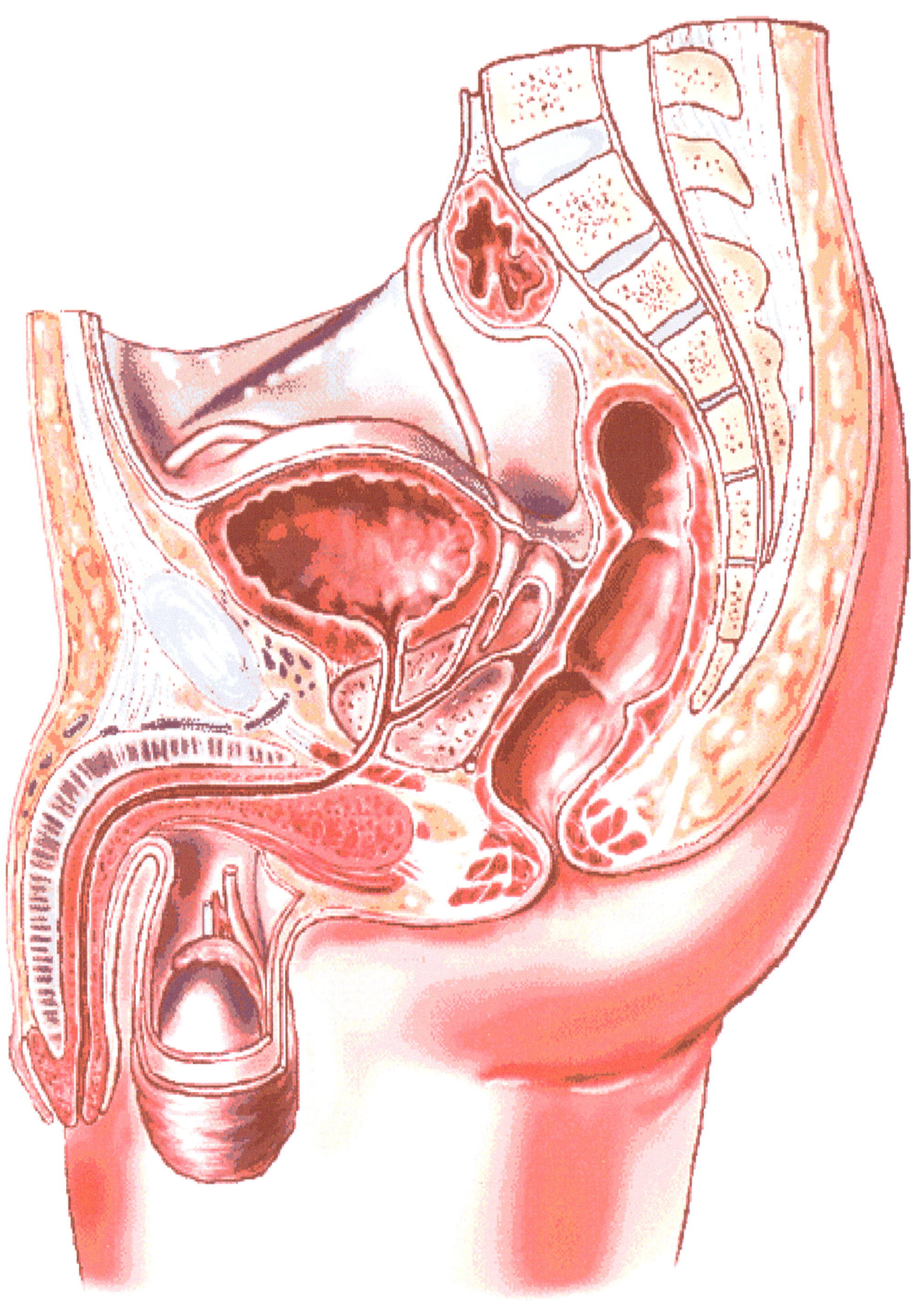

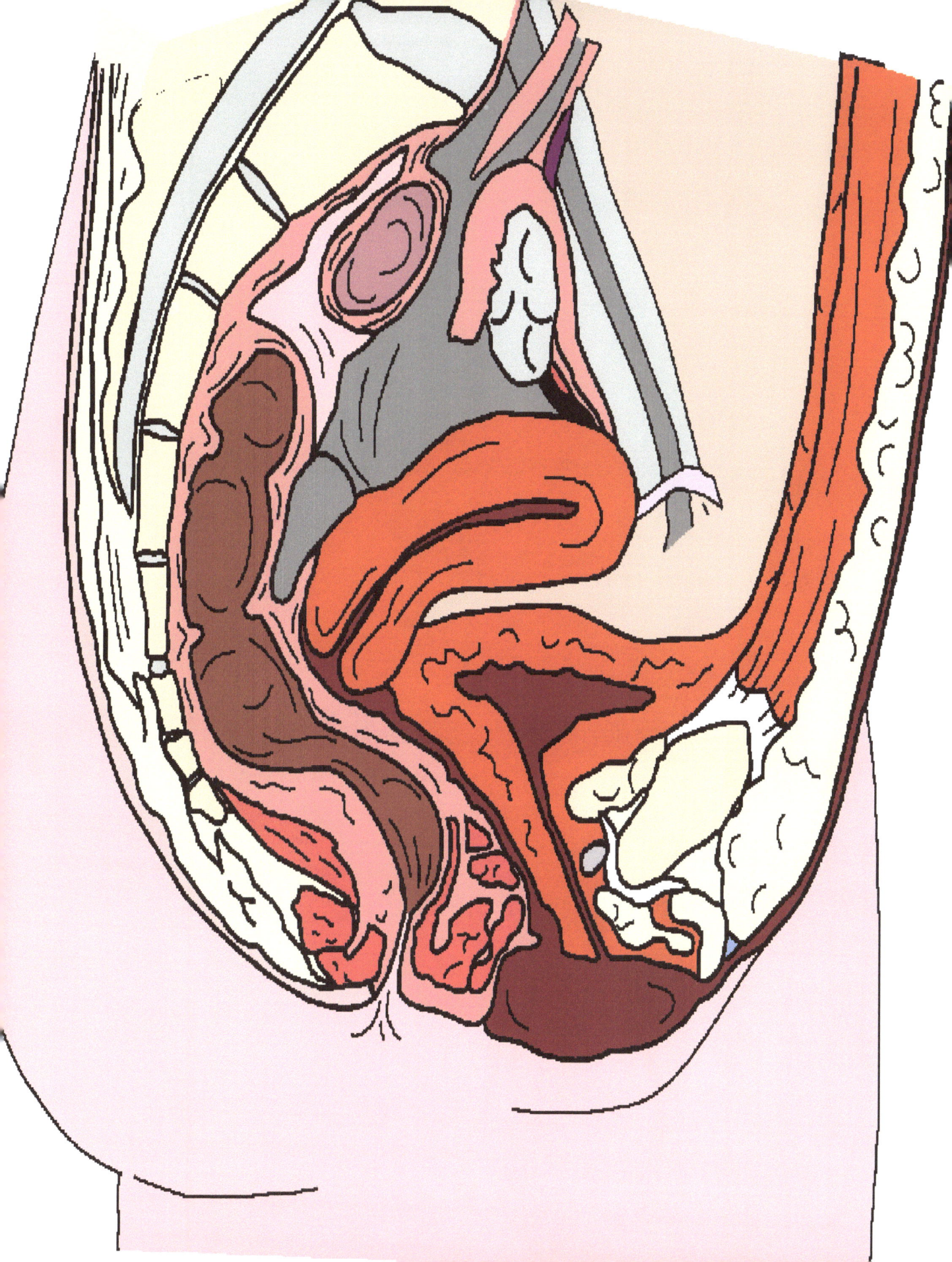

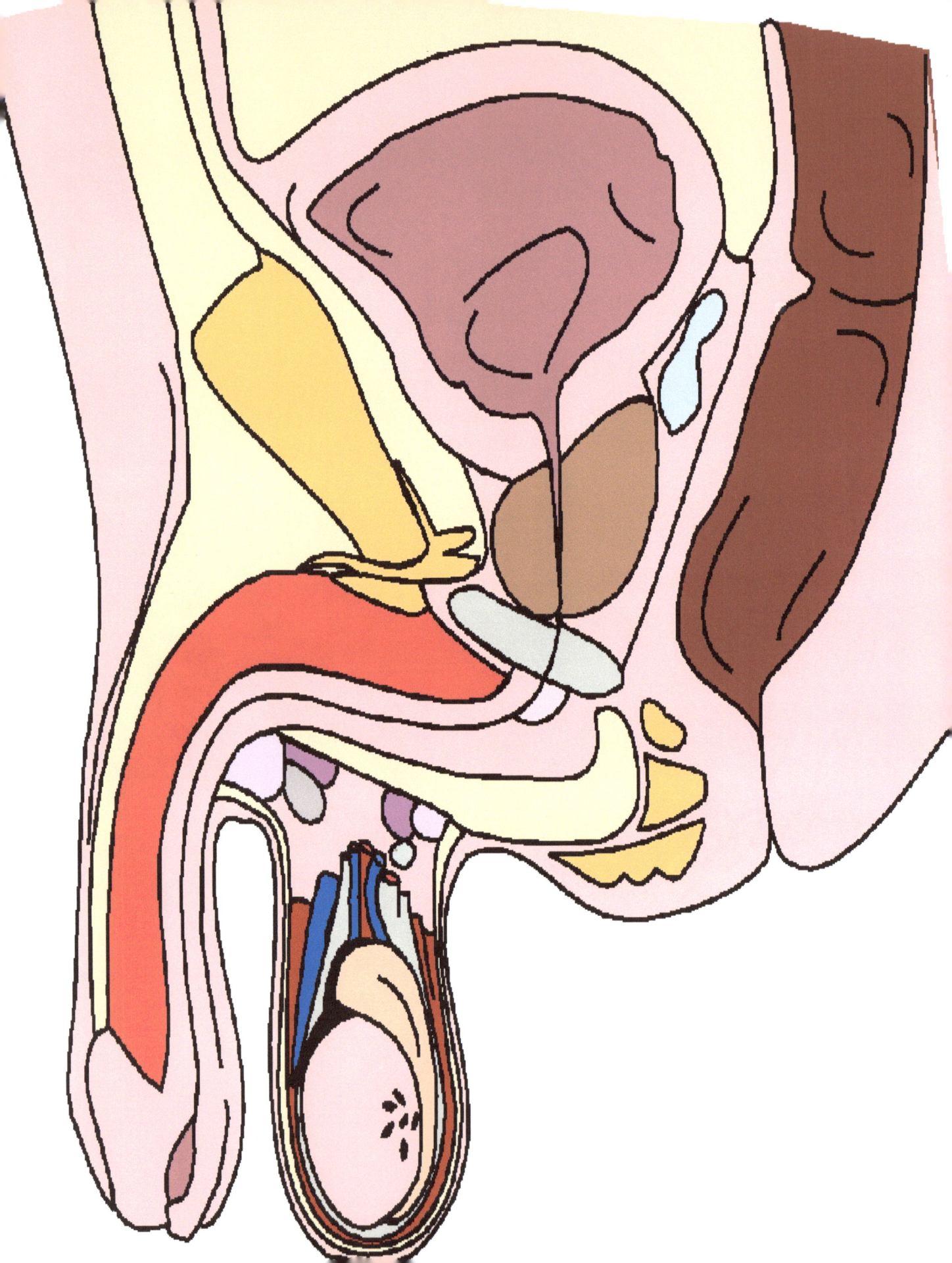

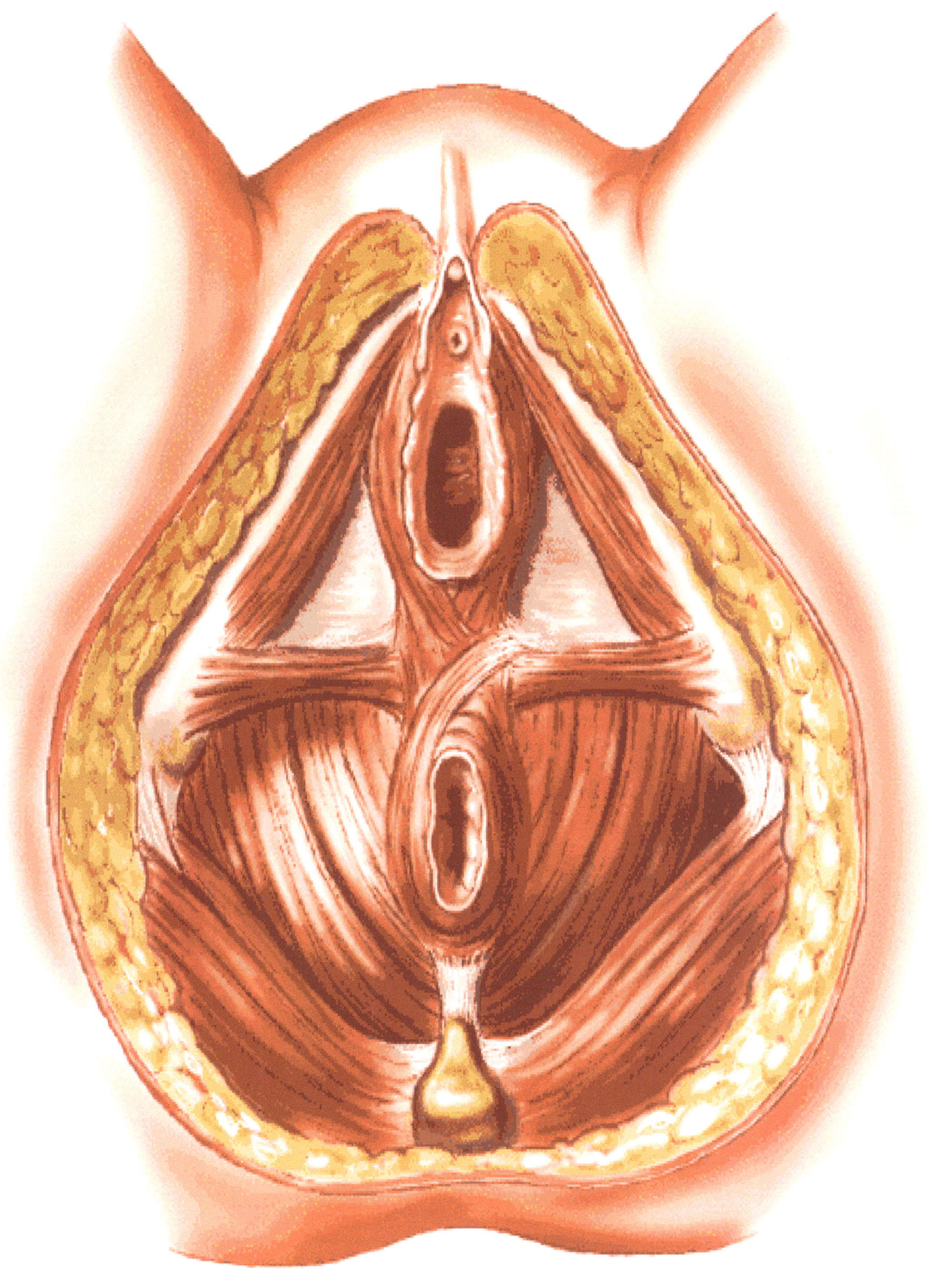

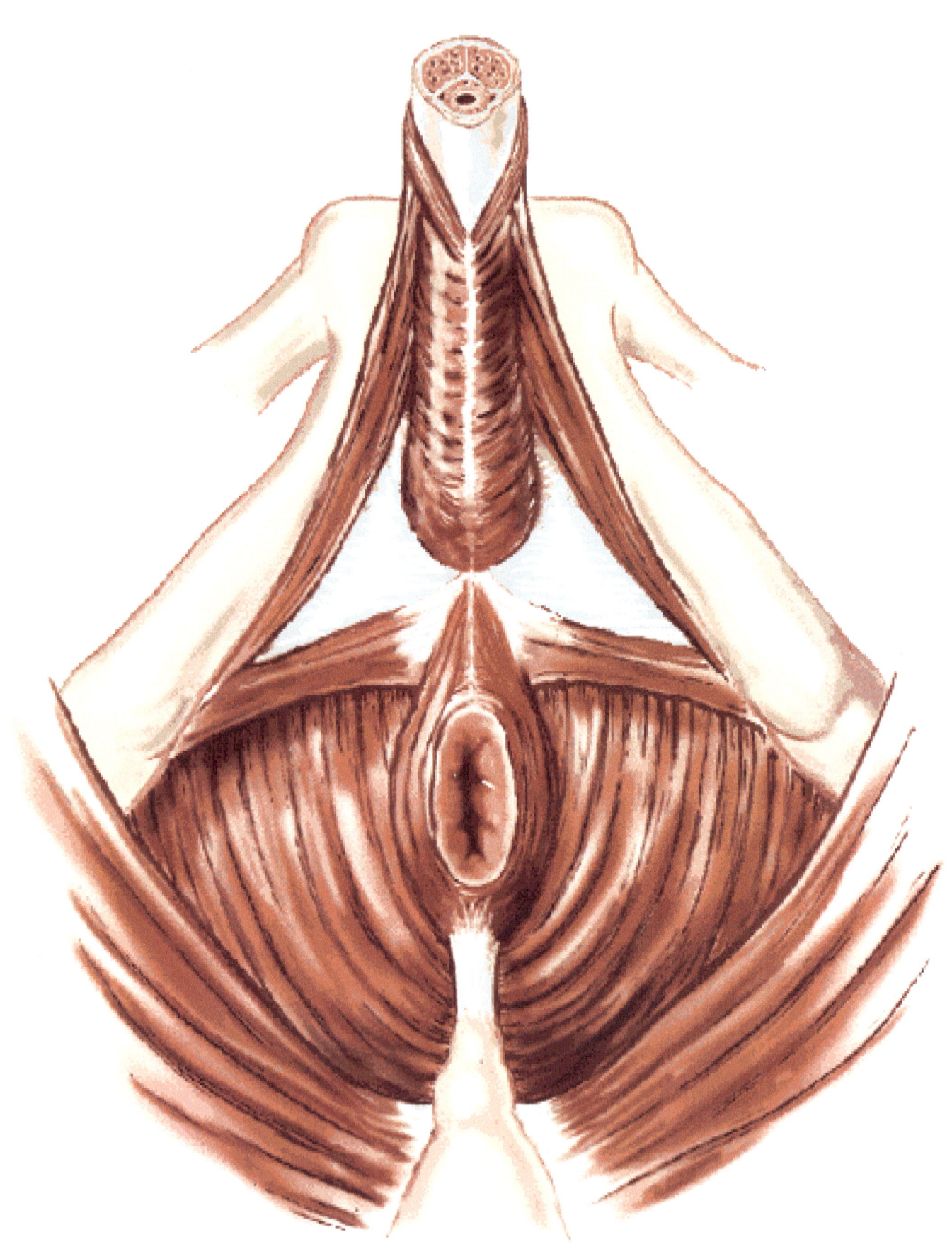

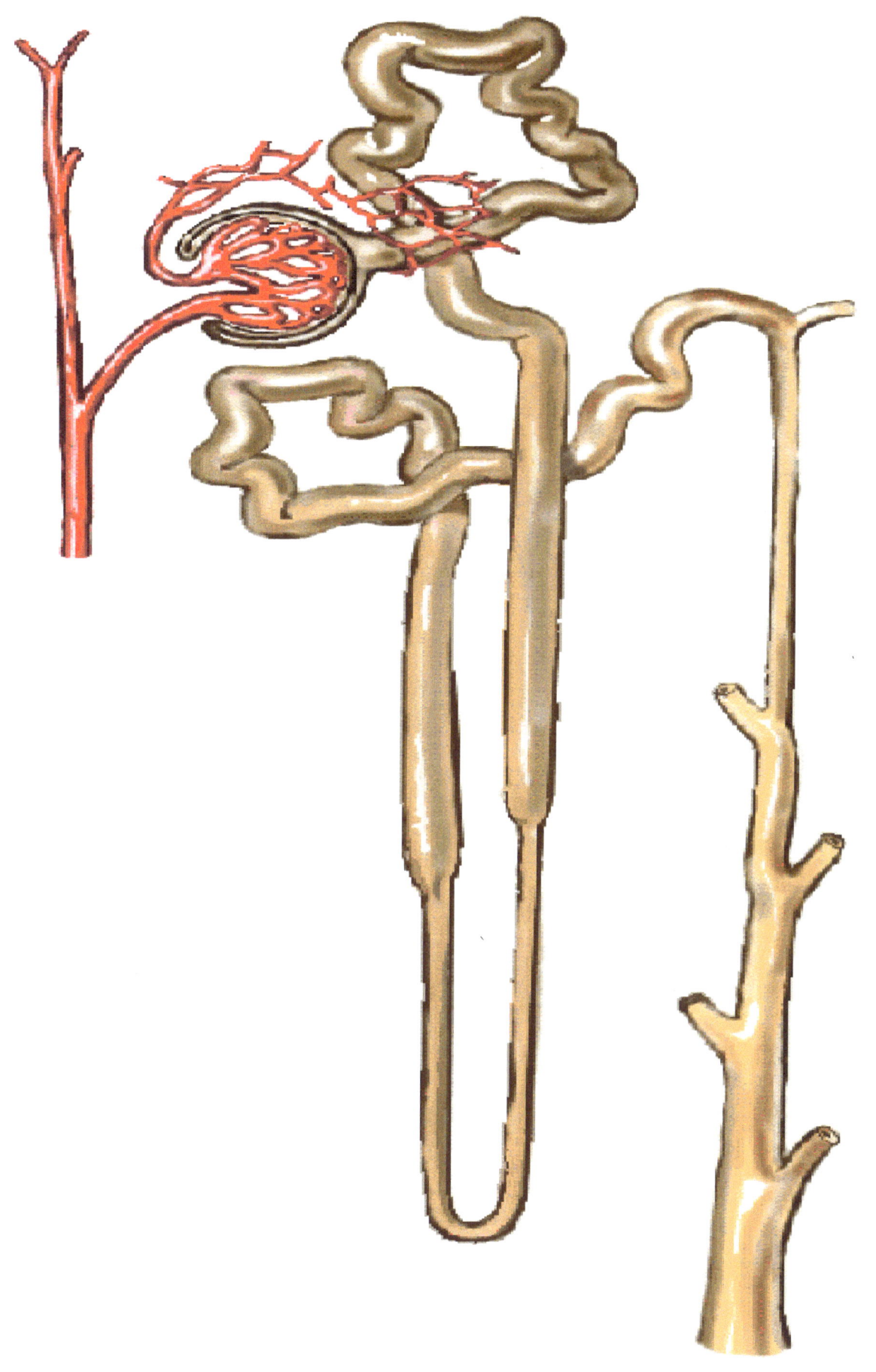

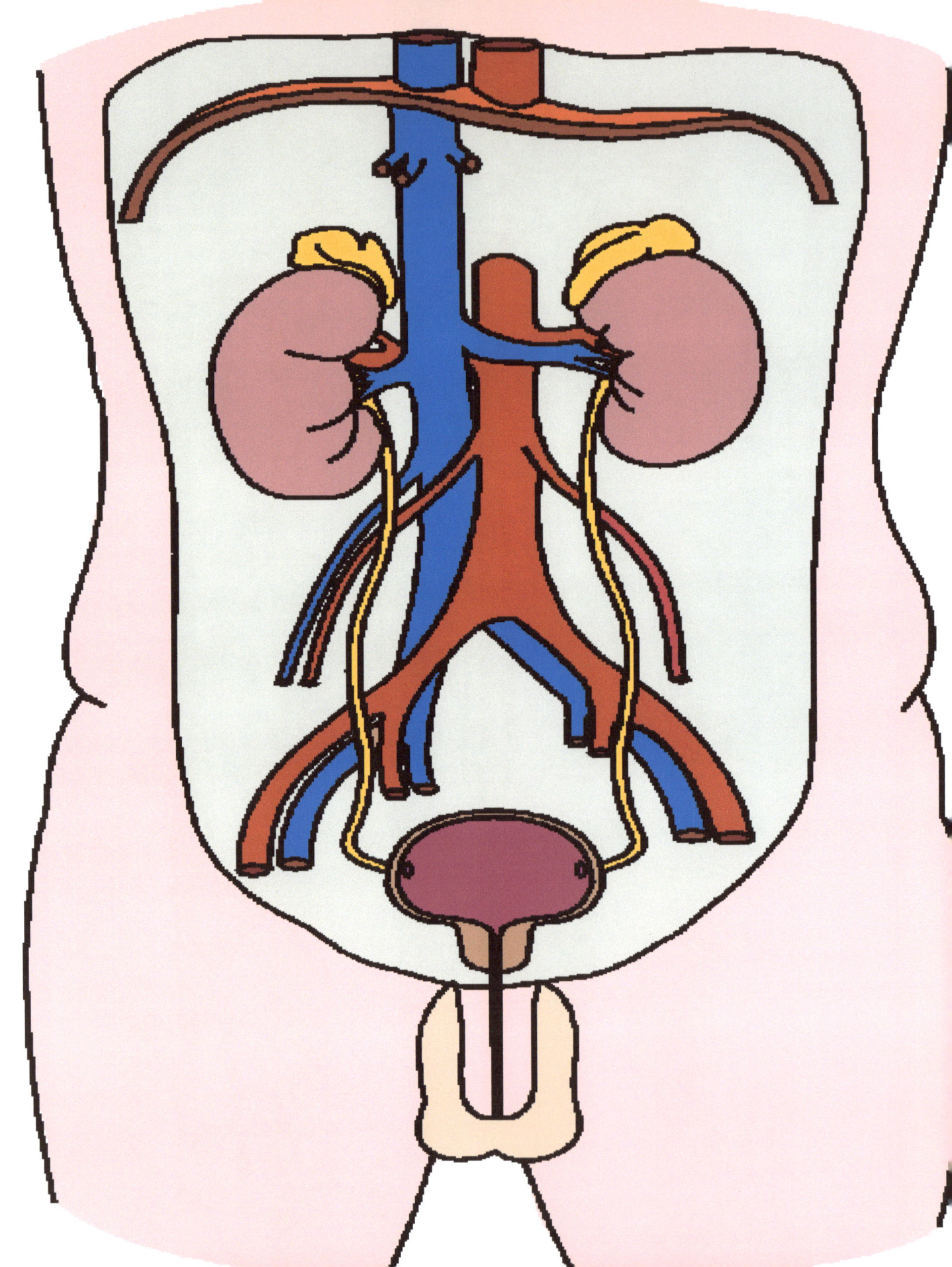

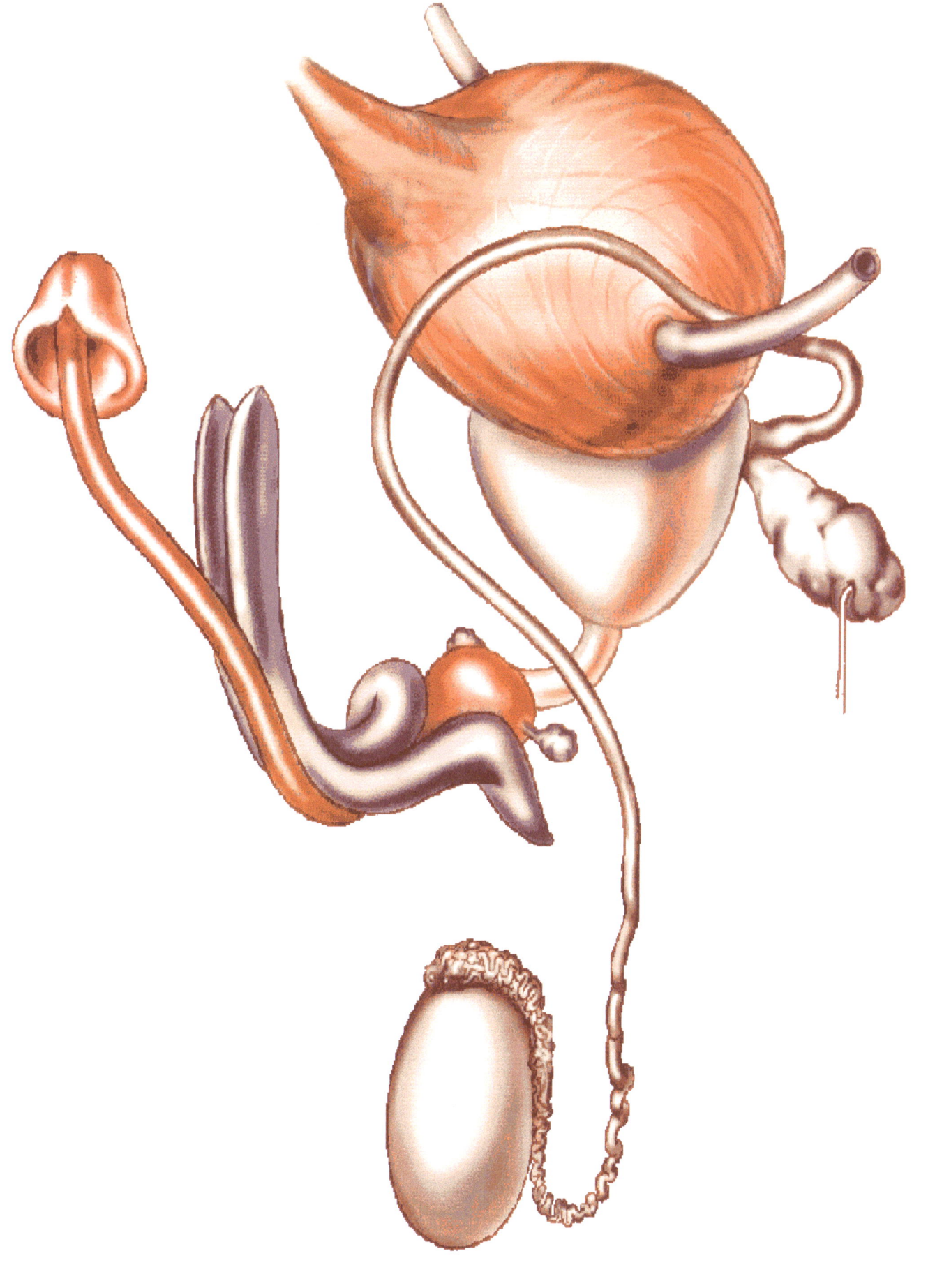

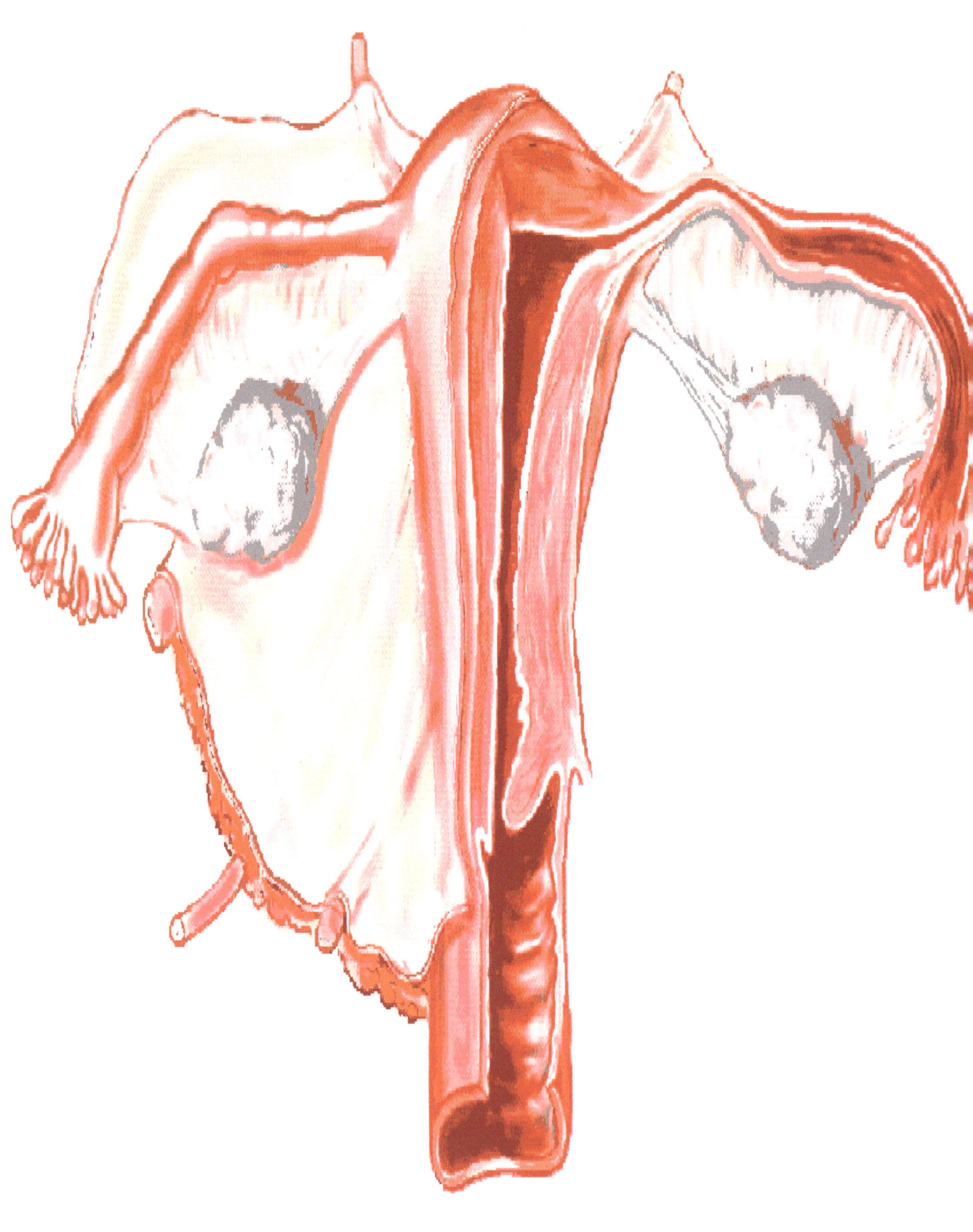

# Other Anatomy System Label Practice Books Available on Amazon

1. Cardiovascular System
2. Digestive & Endocrine System
3. Muscular System
4. Nervous System
5. Respiratory System
6. Skeleteal System
7. Surface Anatomy & Senses
8. Urogenital System

www.ingramcontent.com/pod-product-compliance
Lightning Source LLC
Chambersburg PA
CBHW050415180526
45159CB00005B/2288